Copyright (C) 2013

Breast Massage Secrets Revealed
Special Edition - 3 Books in One

Michelle Tallia

ISBN-13: 978-1490467566
ISBN-10: 1490467564

Erotic BDSM Books - Your Erotic BDSM Book Publisher
EroticBDSMbooks.com

This book comes with two free bonus books (making it a $20.85 total value!) Your books are presented in this order:

Book #1
100 Great Lines to Put In Your Personal Ad

Introduction

The lines in this book can be combined with other lines you may think of to make your personal ad all it can be. Some lines in the book might need adapting to best suit you and/or your sex.

TAGLINES: Your short "tagline" is a headline that, perhaps along with your picture, can get readers to further explore your ad. Great taglines are like gold and people have paid hundreds of dollars for them! Now however many are on the Internet for you to see and use.

Remember, people love to laugh. A funny tagline is a big plus.

There is a great deal of material in this book to build quality taglines from. You may also want to take a bit of time and do a web search for "best personal ad taglines" for ideas. Chances are others (including those looking at your ad) haven't seen the tagline already, or have forgotten it if they did.

This book however is the best collection of personal ad lines that I'm aware of online or offline.

The Lines

A day not in love is a lost opportunity.

My friends know me as spontaneous, spritely, and upbeat.

I am searching for a beautiful person inside and out.

Are you looking for real love and someone special?

I enjoy thought provoking dialogue.

Together let's seek our destiny.

I hope only to fulfill your every desire.

I love making people happy and to see them smile, even if at times it is at my own expense.

I feel the most pleasure when I know I am doing/enduring something to please another.

I'm looking to learn, not just to play....

I'd like to explore hidden fantasies with you.

I want to be taken to that special place and beyond.

I have the financial and emotional capacity to take care of myself.

Unlike perhaps others here I'm not misrepresenting myself. I know the importance of honesty.

I love sex. Rough sex, fun sex, emotional sex... I want you to respect me before and after but during is negotiable.

I want to explore my naughty side,

I'm looking for a friend, confidant and lover.

Like me I'd like you to be thoughtful, attractive, and looking to expand yourself as a person.

I have developed intricate pleasure techniques which can slowly arouse and pleasure beyond imagination.

I think I would describe myself, briefly, as quite a sociable person with a good sense of humor who doesn't take herself too seriously...having said that I believe I am also thoughtful and caring and someone who places great value on good friendships and relationships.

I am loyal, compassionate and respectful of people and animals.

People describe me as easy going and good natured.

I have got great plans and goals in my life which I want to achieve.

I'm a contemporary yet spiritual soul in search of his charming, compassionate and caring companion to share this journey of life.

Are you looking for someone to grow with and push things further?

I have a wise mind and younger spirit.

I am an easy going, and loyal friend.

I'm looking forward to a fantastic voyage of a relationship.

I am attracted to someone who enjoys learning and growing.

Are you looking for fun, adventure and a challenge? If so I'm your girl.

I'm a passionate person with interests numerous and diverse.

I am trustworthy, affectionate, passionate, loving and non-judgmental. I am happy with myself and my accomplishments.

I want someone kind, loving, honest, communicative and self-aware. Your developed interest in education, hygiene, aesthetics, style and emotional literacy would make life easier for us. I'd like to find someone interested in building a relationship based on an accomplished life and a win/win attitude.

I am looking for someone who can work themselves deep inside my mind and make me fall to my knees.

Are you looking for someone to make you happy...someone that won't just have sex with you but will make love to you?

We all want to achieve heart pounding serenity.

I am looking for something more than just sex and games. Sure sex is a part of it but I also want someone that I can spend time with. I want the total package.

I want someone that I can go out with, talk with, laugh with, and fall in love with.

Outside of our playtime, I'd like to enjoy a harmony that can grow into a loving, trusting relationship. I enjoy the outdoors and staying healthy, going out on the town from time to time and hanging out at home.

My last relationship ended because we grew in different directions.

I am usually lucky and love life. I would like to find someone like that.

I'm a strong, seductive, passionate woman who is established and knows herself.

I'm well educated and well-travelled. I'm gainfully employed and very independent. I enjoy traveling, good food and wine, the theater and sports.

I'm searching for an open minded man with an adventurous soul and sensual heart. A journey in love is the destination. We still have plenty of time but none to waste! A beautiful world is waiting. Let's enjoy while we can!

I'll laugh at your corny jokes.

I'm a writer and voracious reader. I'm smart, and I like smart people.

Physical attraction leads to animal instincts.

I have a strong passion for the exploration and power of touch in all its forms.

I enjoy knowledge, I like to learn new and exciting things.

I am cosmopolitan and highly educated. I am a baby boomer, in good shape and would like an agemate and a partner who understands mutuality. I am interested in developing a long term relationship.

I am interested in meeting someone who is honest, open and enjoys (his) her kink.

I have very many interests and I'm passionate about all of them! I love movies, literature, music, art, theatre, science... and lots of other things.

I am fun, open-minded, spontaneous and down for raunchy action.

The reason openness is important to me is that it shows that someone accepts themselves.

I'm lively and active and have a well developed sense of humor.

I hope to always be me and take advantage of any opportunities and chances whenever they're thrown at me.

I am totally devoted when in love.

I'm a laid-back, drama-free kind of person.

I want to be late to my own funeral.

Physical play is quite enjoyable but chemistry and a connection is more important.

I like to laugh, I like to have fun.

I believe that love is not what we see but what we do.

I won't ignore you or abandon you. I'm not looking for a secondary relationship.

I have a well developed and dominant sexual identity. I am seeking a man who is a smart, uninhibited, challenging partner.

I consider myself a natural leader, an innovator, a creator. I fight for the best and readily take the risks incumbent with leading a fulfilled, enriched life.

I am a strong, confident thinker, with a secure sense of himself (herself).

I consider myself to be a spontaneous, fun loving person. I work hard, play hard, and enjoy life. I'm a very affectionate and passionate. I like to hold hands and believe it or not cuddle. I believe in treating others the way I would like to be treated. I am looking for someone to grow with spiritually, mentally and physically. I want someone who is not afraid to love and be loved, someone who is affectionate, passionate and good kisser.

I will love you and take good care of you. I am someone who you can trust and believe in, someone who will always want to make you feel happy.

I'm neat and clean both internally and externally.

I want true love and real commitment.

I am looking for something more than just sex and games. There is a balance that is needed since none of us can live in a purely sexual world. Sure sex is an important part of it all but I also want someone that I can spend time with. I want the total package. I want someone I can go out with, talk with, laugh with, and fall in love with.

I want something that will naturally grow and evolve into its own very beautiful story.

I enjoy a great number of things and am very open to experimentation.

I'm interested in your fantasies.

I want to touch your body, your soul, your life.

I still believe that fairytales can come true, it can happen to us...

I live a healthy lifestyle. I am seeking the same.

I am brimming with sexual desire.

I will be looking forward to hear from you and Your wish will always be done...

I am looking for a partner - but I am happy to form a friendship.

Living on earth is expensive...but it does include free trips around the sun.

I eat healthy and workout regularly.

I am an educated, intelligent professional with eclectic tastes in most everything: art, music, food, people, entertainment and travel.

I'm looking for a non-smoker to share my life with in all ways, a friend and companion to travel with, commiserate over bad days and rejoice over good days; a lover and confidant.

Educated, professional and kinky.

I have class and style. I know the value of dressing to impress.

I would love to be able to say "I've finally found you."

I believe that we all have the ability to create or change anything.

I consider myself to be a sharp, crafty, inventive, fun, strong woman who enjoys life more when she's in a relationship.

I'm looking for a like minded man to chat, debate and play with.

I'm not a just fantasist wasting your time.

I am people biased not gender biased.

I am family-oriented and have family values.

I possess confidence but take pride in not being arrogant. I'm persistent but respectful. I have intelligence and charm.

I don't like negative people. We're here to live life not fear it.

I have learned in life that the smallest good deed is better than the grandest good intention.

I have high hopes for us.

I am a sharp, crafty, inventive, fun woman who doesn't hate men or hate anyone for that matter.

I enjoy life so much more when I'm in a relationship.

What you are like OUT of bed makes you more desirable for me to want you to take me there.

I like to please as much as be pleased.

I want to discover and explore my limits as well as push them further.

I like intellectual conversations.

My ambition is self-actualisation, to release the potential within.

I'm thoughtful, devoted, industrious, competitive, genuine and trustworthy.

I'm looking to learn and grow, not just to play....

The End

Book #2 - Breast Massage Secrets Revealed: Get Pleasure Like You've Only Imagined

Author: Michelle Talia

Copyright (C) 2013

Breast Massage Secrets Revealed

The specialized breast massage discussed in this book can give a woman more pleasure than she can imagine. If her lover is unavailable to pleasure her this way, women can easily give themselves *Extreme Pleasure Breast Massage*, and the great news is it's something women can do to themselves for the rest of their lives.

There are a great many positions a woman's body can be in to receive this specialized and very sexually arousing breast massage. For this example though, let's have her sitting up and at least topless. Do note however that as she gets more and more aroused, she'd probably prefer to be naked so one or both of you can access her pubic area with fingers or toys while she's getting Extreme Pleasure Breast Massage.

For this position the massager sits behind her and up against her back. If it's okay with who is getting the massage, I suggest the massager be naked as many women will lose control at some point when getting Extreme Pleasure Breast Massage and be anxiously reaching behind their lower backs to play with the massager's privates. If a woman has never experienced this type of erotic massage before, she in particular may react with callous abandon.

Before placing yourselves in any of the massage positions, you'll need to have readily available a good supply of quality lotion and/or massage oil. If using lotion, try to use some brand of non-desensitizing lotion. (Most lotions put desensitizers in them to dull the pain of dry skin and other irritations. These desensitizers can at least partially desensitize breasts thus cutting down on the breast's capacity to provide pleasure. Various hair conditioners can also work.) Cold lotion, massage oil or hair conditioner on breasts can provide an unwelcome jolt so if warming is necessary, warm the lotion/oil up ahead of time using the microwave oven, or by setting it in hot water. You can also rub blobs of it in your hands to warm it up. Always have an ample amount of this massage oil or lotion nearby as well as small towels to wipe the oil/lotion off of your hands and her breasts after the massage is over.

Put a sizeable glob of massage oil/lotion on each of your hands, rubbing it all over the palms of your hands to spread it out, as well as warm it if it's not yet warm. Then put your well lubricated hands on her breasts, *but not yet on her nipples and areolas*. This is because those provide the most pleasure and thus the best is saved for last!

It is so important that the massager make sure to keep his/her massaging hands *very* well lubricated. When the oil or lotion is breaking down the massager will feel stickiness developing. The rule of thumb is that you can't lubricate your hands and her breasts too much!

Also the massager needs to make sure his/her nails and skin of their hands are smooth. Trim and file your fingernails and that kind of thing, to as short and smooth as possible. Otherwise she (the person receiving the massage) might feel them as they rub against her sensitive skin. She can even get hurt by them because as she is in the thongs of ecstasy, she might not realize that they are hurting her, so make sure to watch out for her and take care of this situation.

Typically the massage will provide three levels of pleasure. Massaging the fleshy part of her breast (but not massaging her areolas and nipples) should give her pronounced and very welcome pleasure; of course the faster her breasts are massaged the more pleasure she'll get. Including her areolas in the massaging will increase her pleasure a lot. But massaging her nipples will really get her going.

Below (and not in order of importance) are suggestions to optimize the breast massage.

* Start from the bottom of her breasts (where the breasts meet her torso) and work your way slowly higher up to just below her areolas. You can move your hands at varying speeds but typically the faster you massage the more pleasure she'll get.

* Simultaneously circle her boobs with each hand. Start out by using limited pressure on the breasts while utilizing only one finger, then gradually work your way up to utilizing all your fingers. Go clockwise then counterclockwise (or vice-versa.) Remember, *leave her nipples and areolas alone as much as possible until she's practically (or literally) begging for you to*

massage them. Sure you will "bump" into them from time to time as you massage around them. Those bumps will give her a delicious taste of what's to come.

* At its base, wrap each hand around a single breast then run your well lubricated hands around and along that breast in a steady spiraling motion up the breasts in the direction of her nipples, until you reach the edge of her areolas. Of course you can go in the opposite direction also (starting from just below her areolas and working your way down to where her boobs meets her torso.)

* Place one hand on the base of one breast; the back of the hand should be facing her head. Put your other hand on the base of her *other* breast, the back of it should be facing her legs. Slide your well lubricated hands from left to right and then vice-versa, across and along both breasts.

* At its base, take each breast in a well lubricated hand and with increasing speed pull up from the base of her breast to the nipple until your fingers reach the edge of the areolas (or if you're already playing with her areolas and/or nipples, go all the way to her nipples.) Then do the opposite and slide your hands back down from the top of her breasts to the breast's base (where you started from.) Repeat this procedure many, many times.

* Tease her by sliding only your well lubricated fingertips over her breasts, wiggling your fingers.

* Instead of the above, perhaps for a minute or more, you'd like to start the festivities by teasing her breasts by only briefly touching them here and there using only the tips of your fingers.

* Concentrate your efforts on only one well lubricated breast; wrap both hands around it, kneading it, pulling it and twisting it.

As previously discussed, it's strongly suggested that you take your time before playing with her areolas and then nipples. This is because she will still get a good deal of pleasure from having the 'areola and nipple-less' massage. I for one require that she even beg you to play with her nipples--because as we know this is where the breasts offer the most pleasure. I would suggest waiting until she is already well stimulated. You may stroke her anticipation by whispering in her ear that you're about to play with her nipples, then suddenly do it. She may scream with delight as an orgasm overcomes her.

Playing with her nipples is typically the high point of her massage. She'll likely be getting the most pleasure now. (Again, the faster your well-lubricated fingers move around her nipples, the more pleasure she's likely to get.)

Okay massagers you now have a choice, you can immediately start massaging her nipples fast and hard, driving her crazy, or start massaging them slowly, then progressively massaging them faster and faster until she screams in ecstasy. If you're going to massage them fast immediately, as is the first option, many women will start their orgasm then (if they haven't already.)

Don't forget you can let her use a vibrator on herself as you massage her and thus it's suggested you keep a vibrator within arm's reach. Believe me she'll find it if it's there.

Because so often the woman you're massaging will get so aroused from all this that with both hands she'll instinctively reach around her lower back to play with the massager's pubic area. She then will not have a free hand to use the vibrator on herself. Of course both your hands are busy giving her Extreme Pleasure Breast Massage. A way to counter this is to secure a vibrator with white medical tape (the type used to hold gauge and cotton to cuts etc.) over her most sexually sensitive pubic area. (Perhaps it would be helpful if she keeps her panties on for extra support.) If you do this, more women will orgasm while you are giving her this massage.

Remember guys her nipples can get tender after orgasm and need to be left alone for a bit of time.

As is obvious, ladies, you can give yourself Extreme Pleasure Breast Massage in the privacy of your bedroom.

After the massage, ladies your breasts tend to become firmer for a while and often they'll feel quite good for hours.

The following is another way (and quite sexual) of giving this massage. It's told from the perspective of the kinky dominant massager:

I will tell you to stand up and we will go to the bed (if we're not already there.) I will set the bed up so I am sitting with my back against the headboard of the bed and you are laying in front of me face-down on cushions with your head positioned so you can easily suck on my penis and play with my scrotum using your tied-together hands.

Also I'll put a roughly 3' x 3' sheet of plastic under your upper body to keep the massage lotion or oil from going on the bed covers. (More on this massage very soon!)

Perhaps I will also tie your bound hands to the headboard. If I do that though I will make sure there is enough slack in the rope for your hands to still move freely around my penis and scrotum while you suck. If your hands are tied to the headboard, I will be sitting on the rope as my butt will be in-between your bound hands and the headboard which your hands are tied to.

Your breasts will now be positioned, thanks to these cushions, just above the ground. As you suck on my penis, I will generously lubricate (and keep lubricated,) your breasts with some brand of preferably non-desensitizing lotion or massage oil. (Many lotions put desensitizers in them to dull the pain of dry skin. These can at least partially desensitize breasts thus cutting down on the breast's capacity to provide pleasure. Thicker hair conditioners may work also.)

I will warm the lotion/oil up ahead of time or rub it in my hands to warm it up, if warming is necessary. I will then massage your breasts. I will continue for a long time to massage your lubricated breasts as you suck on my penis. (This is known as "Extreme Pleasure Breast Massage". Remember to always keep the massager's hands well lubricated! The two of you will quickly notice that the nipples respond with the most pleasure from this massage.)

You young lady will be required to get a great deal of pleasure from all this which you almost certainly will have no trouble doing. You will have no more than 60 seconds to start orgasming after I first start playing with your breasts in this manner.

Using a yardstick type implement, I can reach across your back and spank you as you suck. Obviously one should make sure the woman can handle being spanked while sucking. Most can depending on the intensity of the spanking and how hard she's already orgasming.

The End

Legal Notice: In this publication there may be inadvertent inaccuracies including technical inaccuracies, typographical inaccuracies and other possible inaccuracies. The writer and publisher of this publication expressly disclaim all liability for the use or interpretation by others of information contained in this publication and/or listed Web sites. The author, publisher and distributors of this publication hereby disclaim any and all liability for any loss or damage caused by errors or omissions, (should these exist) whether such errors or omissions resulted from negligence, accident, or other causes. If legal advice or other expert assistance is required, the services of a competent professional person in a consultation capacity should be sought. the information contained herein may be subject to varying state and/or local laws or regulations. All users are advised to retain competent counsel to determine what state and/or local laws or regulations may apply to the user's particular business. The Purchaser or Reader of this publication assumes responsibility for the use of these materials and information. Adherence to all applicable laws and regulations, federal, state, and local, governing professional licensing, business practices, advertising, and all other aspects of doing business in the United States or any other jurisdiction is the sole responsibility of the Purchaser or Reader. The Author and Publisher assume no responsibility or liability whatsoever on the behalf of any Purchaser or Reader of these materials. Any perceived slights of specific people or organizations are unintentional. Products, services and websites' content vary with time. Please verify any published information.

Book #3 - Absolutely Essential Tips For Buying & Selling On eBay

*eBay is a registered trademark of eBay Inc.

Copyright 2013

Absolutely Essential Tips for
Buying & Selling On eBay

Important Tips for Buying on eBay

1) Last Minute Bidding Frenzies - Perhaps you've noticed that often there's a bidding frenzy in the last one minute of bidding. New bidders may suddenly start bidding in the hope that the previous bidders will not be watching or can't increase their bid in time. Often however it's because of *Sniping.*

Sniping websites automatically bid on your behalf, often in the last 10ish seconds. Simply sign up, enter an eBay item number and the maximum price you're willing to pay. Hidbid.com and goofbid.com offer sniping services that place bids for you.

Typically you'll need to give sniping sites your eBay password for them to work (ugh!!) Obviously that is a serious security concern.

There's little protection from eBay if things go wrong when sniping, since you willingly gave your password to a third party. If you do sign up for such a service, never use the same password for eBay as you use for other accounts like banks accounts or email addresses.

2) Second-chance Auction Scams, Beware of Them - Unscrupulous people sometimes watch bidders in high-dollar auctions and try to take unsuspecting buyer's money after an auction ends.

The scheme, known as a *Second-chance Auction Scam*, is just one of many types of Internet auction frauds reported to the *Internet Crime Complaint Center,* or *IC3.*

Second-chance scammers wait until auctions end and then offer bidders that lost, a phony second chance to purchase the item -- usually through a wire transfer service. This happens more often than people realize, beware!

3) Misspelling Search Tool - Typojoe.com, goofbid.com, bargainchecker.com, fatfingers.co.uk and baycrazy.com - There are many items listed on eBay every day that have misspelled words in the title. It's unfortunate for the seller but chances are good those listings will not come up well in eBay's search engine (because misspelling causes keyword problems) and thus not bring the seller top dollar. Their loss can be your gain!

4) Bidding Tip - Often sellers start auctions at .99 cents, (or at least under a dollar) hoping a bidding war will erupt. Many items go unspotted, staying at this super-low price (99 cents). *LastminuteAuction.com* hunts for eBay auctions due to finish within an hour but where the price still is very low.

With these items in particular, double-check delivery charges, as some sellers hope to recoup costs by charging a little extra (though eBay's now set maximum delivery charges for many categories).

5) Don't Forget About Facebook - *Facebook Marketplace* is a force to be reckoned with. Also sellers often are open to haggling. Just log on to your account at Facebook and search for "Marketplace". It's also worth checking to see if there's any local Facebook selling groups in your area.

6) Nigerian Type Scam for Paying. These unscrupulous people want to pay with a money order that they claim to already have handy. Often it's for more than the purchase amount. He writes to ask if the seller would be "honest enough" (or something of that nature) to send him the extra cash along with the item. (However he might just try to only buy the item with it and not ask for extra cash.) Unfortunately the money order can look okay but is counterfeit. They particularly like the *Buy It Now* feature.

7) Set Long-term Alerts For Rare Items - If you want something very specific or hard to find, set a 'favorite search' and eBay will email each time a seller lists your desired item.

Simply type a product in eBay's search bar, such as "silver dollar", and click 'save search'. Be as specific as possible for the most accurate results. When (and if) someone lists one, you're alerted with an email.

8) Don't Assume eBay's the Cheapest Place To Get Your Item - Many people assume that if it's on eBay, it's automatically the least expensive place to get it, but that often isn't the case. Perhaps you'd also like to use *shopbots* (shopping robots) that check numerous Internet retailers to find the best price. Type into a search engine "shopping comparison sites".

The same rule applies when buying used merchandise. Check used marketplaces on Amazon.com and Play.com - you may even get it for free on Freecycle or Freegle.

9) Check the eBay Going Rate For an Item - There's a quick way to check an eBay product's average price. Enter the item into the search box and click "completed listings". What will come up is a list of prices that similar auctions have already settled on. After that, sort it by "Price: lowest first". If the price is red, it means no one bought it. Green means it sold. Figure out the average price.

10) eBay has banned the selling of intangible items, and that includes curses! - Among the items that were prohibited as of August 30, 2012, are "advice; spells; curses; hexing; conjuring; magic; prayers; blessing services; magic potions; healing sessions; work from home businesses and information; wholesale lists, and drop shop lists."

11) Haggling on eBay Can Pay Off - There's nothing wrong with asking for a discount, even if the listing doesn't have the "make offer" indication. Haggling works best on *Buy It Now* listings, or auctions with a high start price and no bids. Also you'll likely do better if you haggle as the auction is coming closer to closing as the seller could start feeling more desperate.

To contact the seller, click on the seller's nickname then "ask seller a question". If you're polite, you'll likely get further. Blunt requests such as "dude, how about $15?" likely won't work out as well. Remember the seller is likely going to lose money doing this so no point in being annoying.

Once you've arranged a deal, try to keep the transaction within eBay. Ask the seller to add (or change) a Buy It Now price. That way you don't lose the usual eBay buyer protection privileges.

12) Other Things to Do To Exploit Sellers' Screw-ups - Some sellers make basic mistakes, leavings goods going for bargain money.

As well as spelling boo-boos, another error is to leave out key details such as shoe size, dress brand, saying a console's an a Wii when the photo shows a Xbox. At this point, many buyers give it up as "too much hassle".

So contact the seller to fill in gaps, but don't ask the question via the item's listing page, (because that way, when the seller replies, eBay lets them add their reply to the main listing, so it's no longer your secret.)

Instead, ask the question via the seller's profile (make it clear which item you're talking about). They might not bother with the extra hassle of adding it to the listing, so you'll be the only one in the know.

Also the seller might not realize how pricy an item he/she actually has.

13) Tool to Track Down Crazy End Times - Listings that finish at anti-social times often get fewer bids, thus sell for less. To locate auctions that finish when fewer people are around to bid on them, use BayCrazy's *Crazy End Time* search. (A lot more on the best times to end your auction in the next section of the book "*Selling on eBay*".)

Check out their auto-bidding tools if you don't want to spend all that time in front of the computer bidding at odd times. Other

BayCrazy.com tools include "unwanted gift" and "ending now" searches.
www.baycrazy.com/search.php?page=nightowl (Baycrazy offers other eBay related opportunities also.)

14) Search Descriptions as Well as Titles - eBay automatically searches seller's titles for results that include your specified keywords. If you're not getting the results you want, try also searching the item's *description* too. (To do this go to Advanced Search.)

For example, imagine you were searching for a REI Jacket. Unfortunately the seller may be selling one but only put "Ski Jacket" in the title however he mentioned "REI" in the description. Include description in your search and then it should then come up.

15) Search Using eBay Boolean Logic - If a seller could describe an item different ways, you can make eBay search for several different ways of describing it at once. Just place "((" at the beginning and enter different phrases individually enclosed by quotation marks, then followed by commas.

So for example, type... (("fishing tackle", "hook", "reel" ...and it will simultaneously bring up listings that contain the words "fishing tackle", "hook" and/or "reel".

16) Add A Few Extra Cents to Your Bid - When bidding, you enter a "maximum bid", and eBay makes automatic bids on your behalf up to your maximum bid.

Don't enter a round number. For example, if a coat is currently selling for $20, and the most you are willing to pay for it is $25, enter a maximum bid of $25.24. If someone tries to outbid you by entering the round number of $25, they will receive an outbid notice. eBay will go your bid, even though it's just 24 cents more.

17) Be Somewhat Skeptical of Feedback - eBay sellers have a feedback rating that acts as a useful guide to previous seller's opinion's of them. As a guideline, look for a seller with more than 98% positive feedback and a high feedback score of at least 30. Also ensure you read their feedback from their *selling*, not just their *buying*. (To see their feedback, click on their username).

18) Seller with Zero Feedback Could be Cause For Concern - Think twice before purchasing expensive items from a seller with zero feedback.

Remember feedback's useful but not infallible. One thing to watch for is traders selling a number of cheap things for $1ish each to build their feedback, and suddenly listing items costing hundreds each.

19) Check to Make Sure You're Bidding on the Actual Item - Sometimes you assume you're bidding for an item on eBay (or any auction site,) when all that's actually being sold is a link to another site selling it. People are not suppose to be able to sell these on eBay but they can fall through the cracks.

Always read the whole description in detail before bidding. Often the catch is hidden in the text at the end – an attempt to protect the seller from any recourse.

20) Scam - Beware of it - It's a red flag if a seller writes "Before bidding, contact me" then asks for a money transfer. Thieves who hijack actual eBay accounts might use this tactic.

21) Scam - Beware of it - Always be worried if you're asked to pay by an instant money transfer service such as Western Union or MoneyGram. Instant money transfer payments cannot be traced and are highly popular with thieves.

22) Sneakily Find Underpriced Buy It Nows - Feel free to hunt for Buy It Now bargains also. Perhaps the seller under-values their item making their price a good deal.

These steals are snapped up quickly. Go to "Advanced Search", select a category you're interested in, filter it to show *Buy It Now* items and sort the results.

23) Always Complain within 45 Days - Under eBay's buyer protection program, 45 days is the most number of days you have to open a case if you're unhappy with your purchase. (There are some exceptions such as tickets for events that are months away.) Read more on eBay's protection policy.
http //pages.ebay.com/help/policies/buyer-protection.html#conditions1

Under eBay's own Buyer Protection rules, buyers are eligible for a refund if the item's "not as described", meaning it didn't match the seller's description. http://pages.ebay.com/coverage/index.html

24) Pay by PayPal - Avoid sending checks and never use money orders. It's much harder for scammers to disappear with your cash when you use eBay's online payment system, PayPal.

Paying this way costs the same as paying by check, but means you're covered by eBay's Buyer Protection program. If an item is faulty, counterfeit or non-existent, you are far more likely to get a refund.

25) Outbid? Don't Give Up On It Yet - Missed out on a desired item by pennies? Don't give up hope. As every seller knows, sales sometimes don't materialize when buyers change their minds or can't come up with the dough. Because of that feel free to send a friendly message such as: "Hi, I've been looking for this poster for years and just saw your finished auction. Please let me know if the sale doesn't come through."

They may send a *Second-chance Offer*, which are sent out by sellers to unsuccessful bidders if the winner fails to pay up. Ask them to relist at an agreed *Buy It Now* price.

26) Know Your Consumer Rights - When buying from a person who makes or sells goods for resale on eBay you often have the same rights as when buying in person from a shop that does the same. This means your goods must be of satisfactory quality and as described.

With private sellers it's buyer beware. Buyers' only rights under law are that the product is fairly described and the owner has the right to sell it.

Under eBay's own Buyer Protection rules, buyers are eligible for a refund if the item is "not as described", meaning it doesn't match the seller's description.

27) Beware of All The Fakes - While eBay has a 'flag and remove' policy to help identify fakes, still plenty fall through the cracks.

If you're buying big-name brands, do your research first. Carefully check sellers' feedback and post on the forum's eBay board to get others' opinions. Be especially wary of overseas sellers or branded items that seem especially cheap.

The more *unprofessional* the photos, likely the better. Thieves often take professional photos from the brands' sites. Legitimate sellers typically take photos of items at home that might not come out as well.

28) Think Twice Before You Give A Seller Negative Feedback - Of course, negative feedback is often justified but have a heart, don't leave negative or even *neutral* feedback without first trying to work the issue out with the seller. Most sellers are good folks who will try to help particularly, as it can mean a lot to their business to stay in your good graces.

Remember eBay users can view the feedback you've left for others, and if you leave a significant amount of negative feedback, they may well decide you're too high of a risk to sell to.

29) Add An Item You're Interested in to eBay's "Watch List" - Want to keep track of an item without bidding on it? eBay lets you add items to a "Watch List", so you can relax knowing you'll get an email reminder within 36 hours of the auction ending. To watch an item, just click the "*add to watch list*" link in the upper part of the item's eBay webpage.

30) Don't Do Private Purchasing - Sellers may suggest you do a deal outside eBay for a cheaper price. If you do you'll likely have less protection if things go bad. You won't be able to leave negative feedback and you won't be protected by eBay's Buyer Protection Plan.

31) Think Safety When Picking Up An Item In Person - The usual precautions apply. If you get to their door and the seller's holding a butcher knife, now's the time to run.

32) Think International - There's bargains to be had on overseas eBay sites. To include foreign auctions in search results, click "worldwide" for location.

Still can't find what you want? Another option is buying directly from *international* eBay sites. The main ones are USA, Canada, Australia, Germany, France and Spain - there's a full list at the bottom of eBay's homepage. Make sure that the item reads "Shipping to: *worldwide*" before bidding as some international sellers only do business with their country's buyers.

Always factor in postage and if applicable, custom fees. Remember that return postage fees could be hefty.

Also what kind of credit card protections will there be? You're often still protected by eBay and PayPal's buyer protections (if you use PayPal), but it's worth investigating. Type in "buyer protection" in PayPal.

33) Don't Forget The Online Classified Ads - Again, let's not assume that because it's on eBay, that's where you'll get the best price for an item. Unfortunately that's often just not the case. Type "tcp classified ad sites" or something of that nature, into search engines. There's also *Freecycle* and *Freegle*. (Those two sites offer free stuff. freecycle.org and ilovefreegle.org.)

Remember, anyone can post on these classified ad sites. If someone asks you to pay by MoneyGram or Western Union, as always be concerned. It's a bad way to pay.

34) Check Other Auction Sites Also - There are other auction sites that can be found through search engines. If you're searching for something specific, it's also worth adding it to your search. *Auctionlotwatch*.com is a useful shopbot for online auctions. Search for an item and it trawls the big auction sites for you.

35) Check Cashback and Voucher Websites - Check cashback websites to see if there's money back available on your eBay purchase. Type into search engines: "cashback and voucher sites".

Cashback sites give you a cut of their proceeds by setting you up with product and/or service providers.

36) eBay has trained teachers that could be in your area. Also see eBay University. Check out:
http://pages.ebay.com/sellerinformation/howtosell/university.html

Important Tips for Selling on eBay

1) Join eBay Forums - Ask questions about anything, selling, buying etc. Great information is posted already and could be of use. Work together as a team. Find eBay and other auction forums by looking those up in search engines. Ebay has forums also. http://forums.ebay.com/category/Ebay-Discussion-Boards/2001

2) eBay Research Tool 1 - To help in your research about selling items, you can go Type into a search engine "best selling eBay items." EBay provides that information.

3) eBay Research Tool 2 - You can use Ebuyers (www.ebuyersedge.com) to just search eBay for items as well as set up a saved eBay search (or a number of them). You'll get alerted with an e-mail when a matching item is listed.

4) Sell Refurbished Products - Refurbished products fall somewhere in between new and used products. Refurbished products are not new, but often they aren't significantly used either. Sometimes a customer buys the product and for whatever reason, returns it for a refund. The item is then returned to the manufacturer, given an inspection, repaired as necessary and sold as refurbished.

There are various ways an item can become refurbished.

1. The packaging of an item can be damaged during shipping. In that case the item is sent back to the seller/manufacturer. Refurbished items usually come with manufacturer's warranties. Although sometimes the warranties that come with refurbished items are for a shorter period of time, the products are usually in very good condition.

2. Items that have a slight defect or flaw, like a scratch or mechanical flaw, might be returned to the manufacturer. The manufacturer repairs the items, repackages them and marks them refurbished.

3. Demonstration units are also considered refurbished, but generally that's when they're returned to the manufacturer, inspected and repackaged.

4. Brand new overstock items can also be marked refurbished.

5. Sometimes it's a situation where only the packaging of an item is opened. It's re-packaged or even just closed up and marked as refurbished.

Refurbished Products Advantages:

a. Refurbished products are significantly cheaper than new products. They also come with warranties, boxes and everything else new products come with.

b. Selling refurbished products is more profitable, even though refurbished products cost significantly less than new products. On eBay (and at other places) refurbished products can sell for the same price as new ones. (Many people buy refurbished products thinking they're buying new ones.)

c. Refurbished products are sometimes new! When you buy a lot of refurbished products they might actually be overstock items or factory overruns. In that case you would be buying new products at a fraction of the price.

Refurbished Products Disadvantages:

a. Refurbished is not new, even though refurbished products can be exactly the same as new ones, people simply prefer new items.

b. Refurbished products are sometimes the previous year's models. If you're selling electronics or computers it could bring the selling prices down.

5) Finding Products To Sell - Unfortunately finding products to sell can be the toughest part of starting your eBay business. Many people end up opting against starting an eBay business because they can't find a good supplier.

a) YELLOWPAGES.COM - www.yellowpages.com. Try this first. Yellowpages.com can find specialized suppliers in your area. Type in "wholesale" into the search box and you will be given a bunch of subdirectories to further explore. Make sure the search is based on a location near you. Next type "wholesale directory" or "wholesale directories" into search engines.

When searching also try inputting keywords such as overstock, salvage, surplus, liquidation, auction, refurbished, refurb, supplier, closeout, wholesale, etc.

b) BUY FROM AN ACTUAL EBAY SELLER. Buy multiple items and get a discount. That discount could be your margin of profit.

c) BUY WHOLESALE LOTS FROM EBAY AND RESALE THEM - Go to eBay and search for "wholesale lot". If you buy a big lot, you could find you profit best by individually selling the items in the big lot.

d) PERHAPS SELL DIGITAL COUPONS. You should be able to get them for free. As of this writing, people are posting that coupons sell well on eBay. If you're selling coupons, you need to mention that your auction is for the time you spend finding, assembling (sorting) and sending the coupons to the buyer rather than selling the coupons themselves. It's illegal to sell coupons and that's why auctions say the payment is for the time to gather and sort them. Still it can take time to find good coupons and first folks need to know where to look.

e) BUY FROM LIQUIDATION COMPANIES - A liquidator is someone that buys overruns from big retailers (Sears, K-mart, Wal-Mart etc.) at a fraction of the wholesale price. Sometimes big stores can't sell everything they have. The stuff they couldn't sell needs to be gotten rid of as soon as possible to make room for new products. This is where liquidation companies come in. They buy the overruns products, often at a fraction of the wholesale price. When a liquidation company buys a couple of truckloads full of overruns, the next thing it must do is sell these overruns ASAP to make room for more overruns. Since the liquidator must get rid of the products as soon as possible, the products are sold at cheap prices and often in bulk. Perhaps there are liquidator stores in your town what would make you a deal and you wouldn't necessarily have to buy in bulk.

f) EBOOK SALES - With ebooks, you can sell a digital product that can simply be emailed to your customer. No packing and shipping involved! Selling ebooks on eBay is easy. In fact there are systems you can implement to essentially automate the entire process. You could do a *Buy It Now* auction, or just start the bidding at a reasonable price. When the auction ends and the buyer pays you, all you need to do is email the eBook to them. Again, that's the great thing about downloadable information products: no packaging or shipping is necessary. Perhaps you'd like to offer an entire collection of eBooks to sell on eBay. You'll need eBooks that you own or have given you resale rights.

g) You can sell peoples' houses, cars, boats, or even jewelry collections. Just look in the for sale listings of your local newspaper and look at all of the great stuff for sale that would sell on eBay. Call up the owners of the items advertised in the newspaper and offer to sell the stuff for them. Looking for stuff in newspapers is great because the people that are using a newspaper to sell something probably know little about eBay and are desperate to get rid of the stuff they're advertising. These people are also the ones that are willing to lower the price and haggle, and that is great because the lower the price they are willing to let the item go for, the more profit you can make by selling their stuff.

h) RUNNING ADS TO FIND MERCHANDISE - You can run ads in print media and/or post what you're looking for in Internet forums with something like "I will buy your stuff". As previously noted, if you are going to use this method you will need to pick a used product that keeps its value well. If you're going to use this method you should buy things like jewelry and watches, antiques and other things that appreciate with age.

A previous seller's success story was selling old collectable Apple computers. This is a type of item that some people have laying around in the basement or attic, and will likely never use again. They're more than happy to unload it and get a little money for it at the same time. But on eBay it was a whole new ballgame. There are thousands of people who collect old collectable computers.

6) Sell To Resellers - Anyone looking to buy products and resell them to make a profit is a very good customer that will come back and buy from you again and again. Plenty of people buy stuff on eBay then resell it on eBay! There are also those who buy products on eBay to resell them on their other ecommerce websites or actual stores they may own. A lot of PowerSellers (special higher volume eBay sellers with a closer relationship to eBay) started by buying stuff off of eBay and simply putting it back up for auction.

7) Order Samples If Possible - This is a particularly good tip if you don't have a chance to inspect and see the products you are ordering in person. Many people starting out on eBay make the mistake of placing a big order before actually seeing what they're ordering. By ordering samples you'll be able to test not only the quality of the products you're ordering but the service, communication and legitimacy of the company you're ordering from. If you're thinking of selling designer clothing on eBay, be extra careful when ordering your supplies from the Internet. There is a lot of fake (counterfeit) clothing being sold on the Internet. Remember the pictures on the supplier's website may look real, but that doesn't mean they will be sending you what's in the picture.

If you find a great deal but the "supplier" won't allow any sample orders and wants you to pay through an untraceable method, be wary.

8) Second-chance Offers - If the buyer of your item falls through, you can send the other bidders a *Second-chance Offer* to see if they're still interested in buying it.

9) The Listing's Title - The title of your listing should be clear, relevant to what you are selling and attention grabbing. Always include the correct spelling of the item in the title. Don't try to make the title "cool" by deliberately misspelling words, unless perhaps if the slang name for it is popular. If you misspell the title, your listing won't show up in search results because presumably most people aren't searching for the slang name (or misspelled version) of the product.

The title has to be short (eBay rules), so make sure you include the name of the item and abbreviated descriptions, and try not to waste any space on words that are not needed. *By the same token, always use the entire allotted space to write your title. In general, the longer the title, the better, as long as all your keywords are relevant.*

10) Keywords & Relevancy - Make sure the brand name of what you're selling is in the title! If you're selling a Champion Portable Generator, your listing title should include the make and model number, in this case "New Champion 42431 Portable Generator, 1500 Watt". Your listing title should be a short, abbreviated description of the item you are selling.

The name of the product in the title has to do with the search results (keywords). If people want to buy your portable generator they may search "portable generator, generator, Champion, Champion portable generator," etc. You want to make your listing show up in as many search results as possible.

In review, a wild but catchy title will definitely grab the attention of most people who see it, but won't come up in many people's search results, unless also in the title listing is the name of the product that people would type in when looking for it. (Even that's not guaranteed to work.)

11) If a potential customer wants other people's opinions on a product you sell, you might want to send them to the Amazon.com's webpage for the site as Amazon posts feedback from buyers of that same product. Make sure that Amazon is not selling it for less than you are or that idea could backfire!

12) Mention Flaws: If there is a flaw in the item you are selling, make sure you mention it (though try to call it something else like "scratch" or "mark" if that's what it is.) If your product has a flaw and you don't mention it in your listing, you could get negative feedback and a request for a refund from the person who buys the "flawed" item.

If possible, make the flaw sound positive. You could say "this product has a small dent that has no effects on its operation, but because of this you save big bucks!"

Mentioning a flaw also can make you look like an honest person. You can even have the flaw mentioned in your bullet points - Small scratch on the top (saves you money!!)

13) Host Your Own Pictures - You can host your own pictures on another website or your eBay Store and thus show many, many more photos free of charge.

14) Payment Options: - You should offer the customer several different choices of payment. Most of your customers will pay you through PayPal, (PayPal is owned by eBay,) so make sure you get a PayPal account (www.PayPal.com). Of course, not everyone who buys items on eBay prefers PayPal, some may prefer Western union's Bidpay or another payment system. Another one you should sign up for is StormPay as it can be used by people in some countries where PayPal is not used or as popular. For your free StormPay account go to: stormpay.com.

Wire Transfers - Unscrupulous overseas buyers prefer these as they're not as traceable. It's preferable not to take them.

15) Offering SquareTrade Warranties - If applicable to what you're selling, another good way to build trust is to sign up for SquareTrade warranties at www.squaretrade.com. www.squaretrade.com/seller-faq

16) About Me Page - The About Me page is often overlooked by many eBay sellers (and buyers.) While having the free About Me page likely will not dramatically increase your sales, it can help if you have good things to say about yourself and a nice picture. Note, many sellers only include links to their listings and maybe not enough information about themselves in the About Me page.

17) People Bidding with 0 Feedback ratings - Having a good to great feedback rating is so important as you know. Many sellers refuse letting members with 0 feedback bid on their auctions. Getting a negative feedback from somebody that unpredictable is simply a risk we don't want to take. In many cases, we simply don't trust them.

18) Best Time To End Your Auction - The best time for an auction to close (end) is in the evenings and on weekends as that's when most people are on the Internet for that type of activity! You want to make sure that when your auction is closing (ending), everyone that's interested in it is available to bid on it. The mornings are the times that the eBay website gets the least visitors (as people are more often sleeping or working.)

If you live in the Eastern Time Zone, list your auction between 9pm-11pm, Central Time Zone list between 8-10pm, Mountain Time Zone between 7-9pm, and for the Pacific Time Zone list between 6-8pm. This will give you the biggest exposure at the end of your auction. The debate is out as to what day your auction should end on. Some sellers report that Tuesday, Wednesday and Thursday are best. Other sellers report that Saturday and Sunday are best.

There are a few exceptions though. For example, some business products sell best during weekdays and during work hours. Obviously this is because people are usually ordering those types of products at work, for work. Studies have shown that a listing that ends at peak hours can attract up to 25% more bids than one that ends in non-peak hours. Listing your auctions at optimal times is one of the easiest ways to attract more bids.

To end the auction in the evenings, you'll need to put the item for sale in the evening (*or use listing software [see next page] to do it for you*) as eBay considers each day to have a length of 24 hours.

Note, it's eBay's practice that when someone's auction is ending, that listing shows up higher on keyword search results (which is a good thing!)

19) Terms of Service Webpage (Yours) - That's something even a lot of experienced sellers don't seem to include, though it likely won't be necessary if all the information is already in your FAQ webpage. For instance, what's the return policy? What are the shipping options, and what will they cost? What are the accepted methods of payment? How soon is payment to be sent? What is the warranty?

20) Listing Software (For Your Items) - Listing software organizes your eBay listings making the listing part of your business simpler and more efficient. There are many different kinds of listing software. You can do an Internet search for them.

Turbo Lister is free software from eBay. Turbo Lister allows you to upload thousands of listings at a time. It saves listings, schedules your listings and uploads them to eBay automatically. Using it you can edit multiple listings at the same time, preview what your listings will look like before uploading them and more. More eBay software is offered at:
http://pages.ebay.com/help/sell/advanced_selling_tools.html

21) Drop Shipping What You Sell - With drop shipping all you have to do is list items up for auction and when they sell, you contact your supplier, who ships the products from their factory, straight to your customers. In theory drop shipping is a good way to go, but it could offer problems. What happens when you sell items and your supplier sends them to the wrong addresses? What happens when you sell items and your supplier is out of stock? In those cases your reputation suffers. If you are going to use drop shipping; make sure there is good communication between you and your supplier (drop shipper.) Also make sure you have some products in stock in case the supplier runs out by the time your auctions have closed.

22) eBay Stores - eBay stores can be great if you have a number of items to sell. First you'll need to reach the minimum number of feedbacks required (10) to open one. Most PowerSellers have eBay stores. Store sellers can see an increase in profit of up to 25% in the first three months of opening the store (according to eBay). Having your own eBay store can save you a substantial amount of money in listing fees and let you sell items in a fixed price format as well as selling via auctions. Also you can list items for a much longer time and store them in your inventory list for 30, 60, 90, 120 days and even "Good till Cancelled". You'll can feature links to other auctions in all your listings by utilizing a cross promotion tool. There are also bonuses like your own search engine and monthly reports from eBay featuring statistics and dada about your sales in the past month.

An eBay store also gives you a location. It gives you a base of operation, a place where people can easily find you, and a place where repeat customers can come back to. Your customers will be able to bookmark and return to your store, and it may also be indexed in the major search engines. So if you're selling silver dollars, and someone does a BING search for silver dollars, your eBay store may appear in the results along with the usual online retail websites! Obviously this can increase your traffic greatly, and likewise boost your sales.

23) Your eBay Store Identity - Ideally your eBay store should look different from your competition. You can use the design templates eBay offer you, but perhaps it's best to use original graphics. Fortunately eBay Stores are customizable. Ideally, to establish your name, your eBay store should appear like your listings as much as possible. Same colors, design and look.

24) Get a Domain Name - You need to get a simple and memorable domain name. A domain name makes it simple for people to find you. The standard web address eBay will give to your store will look like this: *stores.ebay.com/yourname*, this is not a very memorable web address and it's too long to be easy to type into a web browser. It would be best if you had a web address like *mystore.com*.

The End

www.ingramcontent.com/pod-product-compliance
Lightning Source LLC
Chambersburg PA
CBHW071343310526
45790CB00018B/1200